DIY Healing Salve:
20 Organic Herbal Salve Recipes for Healthy Living

The information herein is offered for informational purposes solely, and is universal as so. The presentation of the information is without contract or any type of guarantee assurance.

The trademarks that are used are without any consent, and the publication of the trademark is without permission or backing by the trademark owner. All trademarks and brands within this book are for clarifying purposes only and are the owned by the owners themselves, not affiliated with this document.

Table of Contents

* * * * * * * * * * * * * * * * *

Introduction: A bit of Salve

There is no doubt that we live in a highly mechanized, technological world. But if we could just get away from the tech solutions that have been foisted upon us for a brief moment and get back to some of the more natural remedies that nature can supply we would be surprised at the results. There are several everyday herbs that can be grown right in your backyard that can provide you with tremendous results.

Herbal salves work by modifying medicinal herbs to where their potency is maximized for the utmost healing effect. These salves can be used to treat all kinds of stress, body aches, skin irritation, cuts, burns, and even indigestion. Herbal salves have been used for about 6000 years now and there is no reason for their use to stop anytime soon. In fact, even the professional medical profession has started to take note.

Returning to the roots of early fathers of medicine such as Aristotle and Hippocrates, many modern doctors are having their hospitals and clinics stuck up on herbal salves. You can't go to a burn unit, for example without finding the place completely stocked up on Aloe Vera Salve used to take the sting out of their patient's burns. Healing Salve can also take the sting out of your medical bills since all of the material that is required to make these salves work are very easily and cheaply available.

There has been quite an awakening when it comes to herbal healing, and especially herbal salves. Many are waking up to the fact that not everything can be solved with synthetic chemicals produced in the lab and instead have returned to Earth for that little bit of healing salve that only nature could provide for us. It all simply serves to remind us that just a little bit of Salve can go quite a long way.

Chapter 1: Herbal Salve for your Aches and Pains!

There is nothing worse than waking up in the morning to find yourself with a stabbing pain in your back or aching muscles in your arms and legs. These aches and pains are not only uncomfortable they can be debilitating and great interfere with daily activity. Diagnosed as "Myalgia" (Muscle Pain) doctors have prescribed over the counter pain killers for decades just to battle the normal pains that present themselves as are bodies wear out from age and use.

These drugs can cover up the aches and pains we feel for a short time, but the trouble is, this concealment of our pain is only temporary, and once we develop a tolerance to whatever pain killing drug we are taking, they come to the surface once again. Through the use of natural, healing salves however, those aches and pains can be eliminated from their very root. In this chapter we will go over some of the best of these natural remedies for the elimination of these aches and pains.

Burdock Root Salve

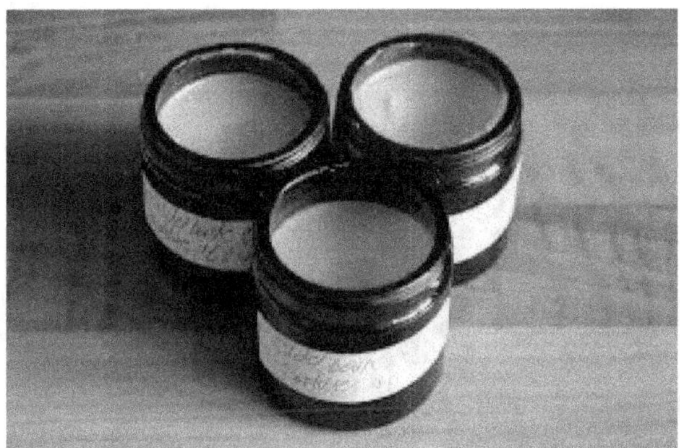

This root has an uncanny ability when it comes to alleviating joint stiffness and pain. This herb can be turned into a salve by grinding it down to a into a fine chalky paste. Burdock Root Salve can then be applied directly to the skin, directly over the aching joint that is afflicting you. The soothing effect of this salve is almost instantaneous. You will feel a slight tingling as the salve begins to work its way into your body.

If you are looking to forage for this plant yourself, to create your own salve from it, the best time to do is in the early summer and late spring. Burdock is known for its pink or purple colorings. Just pull it right up out of the ground and then grind it into a fine powder or paste. After that you can then mix it up with some wax, put it all in a pan on medium heat, cooking the ingredients until they are well melted together. After this store the contents in a mason jar until you wish to apply it.

Valerian Root Salve

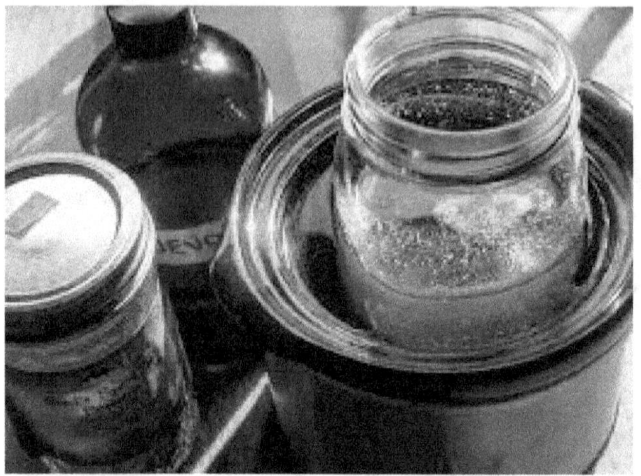

This herb presents us with a truly wondrous salve with multiple uses and benefits. Valerian Root Salve can be used to soothe muscle cramps and leg spasms. Ground down into a powder this salve can be placed directly to the source of your muscle spasms and Valerian root Salve will send a signal to your nerve endings in order to smooth out those cramped muscles and spasms.

Valerian grows naturally in India, Mexico, and Europe, but you don't need a passport to get your hands on this salve, because most health food stores in your local area will no doubt have a well stocked supply. If you purchase Valerian in its pure root form, you should grind it down to a fine powder, and place it in a small plastic container for later use. When you need to apply this salve, simply rub it into your skin. Your muscles should begin to relax and your cramps and spasms will go away.

Devil's Claw Salve

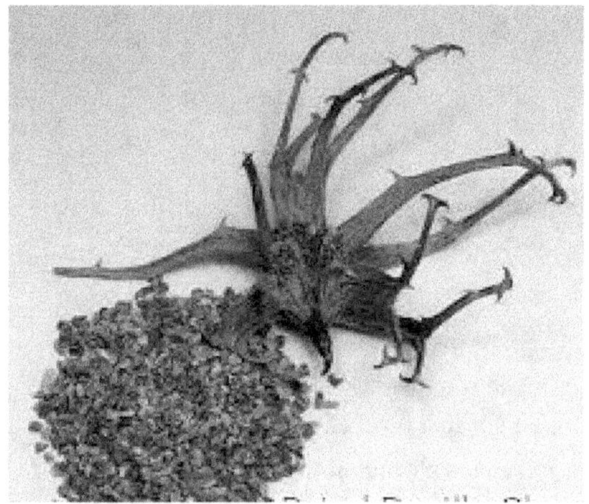

Some approach a herbal salve named after the devil with a bit of trepidation but the healing powers of this salve are a true God send in the way that it can heal our aches and pains. This salve is especially useful for chronic back pain. Simply grind it up and apply as needed. The powerful soothing agents in this herb have tremendous powers of relaxation when it comes to stubborn physical pains in the boy.

So grind up a batch of Devil's claw and put it in a sealed plastic container for those days when you could really need some pain relief! I can remember years ago when I did hard physical labor at a warehouse, I used to carry a small container of this stuff with me in my lunch box, and I can vouch from my own personal experience, that as soon as I applied the material to the part that ailed, the relief was instantaneous!

Turmeric Powdered Salve

You might know this herb as a good ingredient in a bowl of rice, but much more than a tasty additive, turmeric has the power to reduce chronic inflammation. Turmeric contains a powerful acting agent called, "curcurmin" which can be used to soothe arthritic joints and wrists. This herb has been used in this manner for thousands of years. It is great for reducing back ache and stomach problems.

This salve is best in powdered form, or by having it rubbed directly into the skin. This salve being a natural food additive is completely edible and sometimes I consume it direct by eating soup or drinking tea. I have found when I do this it can instantly clear up any aches and pains that I have. Yes, there is more than one way to use a Turmeric Powdered salve!

Ginger Healing Salve

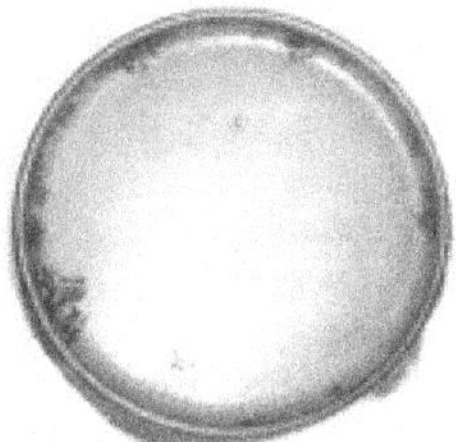

Once extracted and delivered into a salve format the powerful joint and muscle pain relieving ability of ginger is absolutely astounding. Ginger carries special anti-inflammation agents known as "phytochemcials" these acting agents work to reduce inflammation of all kinds. Once your Ginger is ground up into a powder, just rub it right onto the area that is bothering you and you will begin to feel better. Since Ginger is so potent I usually store it in a non descript tin can. But if you have nothing else just find a durable plastic container with a lid. If you are suffering from intense inflammation, then Ginger Healing Salve is definitely worth a try.

Chapter 2: Herbal Salve Immune System and General Wellness

The general wellness of our immune system is of paramount importance. Our immune system is the body's natural filter and protection against the external environment. Think of the immune system as a kind of inborn military barracks that houses battalions of white blood cells that it can unleash at a moments notice in order to destroy foreign invaders. But if your immune health is not up to par the emergency alert system of your body will fail to notify these protective little soldiers of the intruding threat. In order to keep your immune system on guard, there are several Herbal Salves that you should use to keep it up to task.

Cat's Claw Salve

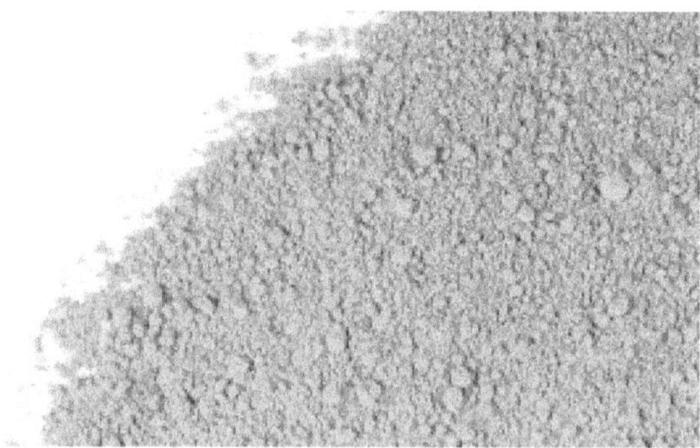

The Cat's Claw is loosely related to the "Devil's Claw" which was mentioned earlier in the previous chapter of this book. In it's herbal form the Cat's Claw plant's curved shape tends to resemble a claw, hence the name "cat's claw". This herb has been used in medicine thousands of years over as an aid in immunotherapy. This herb increases immune system health by giving the body more robust white blood cells, in particular, Cat's Claw works to intensify the special "microphages" within the immune system to make the immune response more rapid and more effective.

As a rapid response system, Cat's Claw can provide the immune health that you need. Cat's Claw Salve has been especially helpful for Cancer patients, who need to buffer some of the effects of Chemotherapy. Cat's Claw Salve can give you the edge you need. Just grind it down into a fine powder and apply it liberally to the chest and arms. Let this salve be absorbed into your skin. You will most likely feel a slight tingling sensation as the active ingredients begin to work their way through your body. You will soon be feeling better in no time.

Astragalus Salve

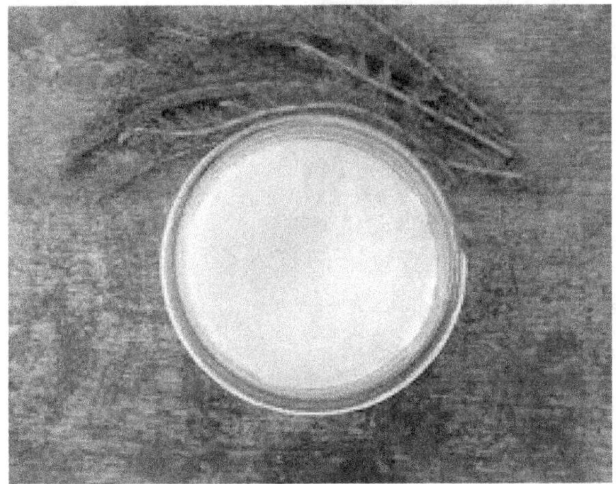

This herb hails from China and has been in use for centuries as an herbal salve. The power of this herb comes from the powder and oil that are extracted from the plant. Whether in powder or oil form, this healing salve can be used to help you fight off severe colds and flu just by rubbing Astragalus Salve on your chest. This salve can also be applied through poultices and wraps.

The first thing that you will notice after being treated with Astragalus is how well it opens up your breathing passages, working partially as an aromatic agent, Astragalus is able to help you breathe while fighting off germs and viruses. This is a mighty salve that also makes for some great skin. Just by rubbing it onto your face it can give your countenance a healthy shine! Don't miss out on this Salve!

Lotus Healing Salve

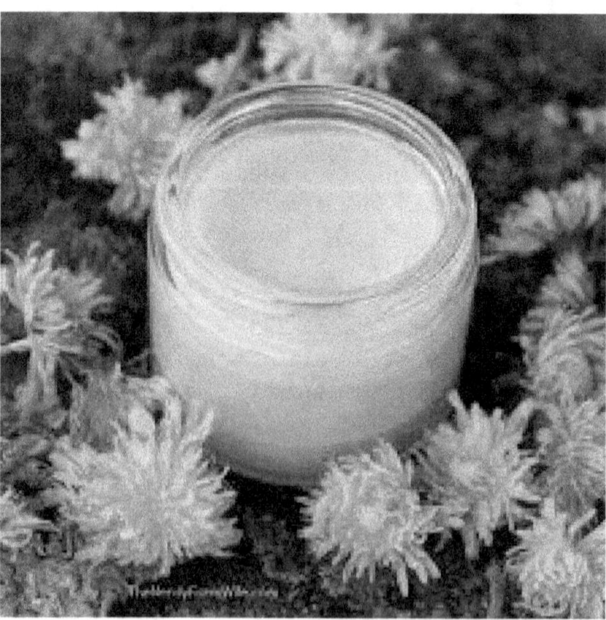

When people think of the Lotus Flower, thoughts come to mind of Buddhists sitting cross legged in meditation. But you don't have to be the Buddha to enjoy the wondrous tranquility of Lotus Salve. The oil extracted from these flowers is what makes up the healing salve from this herb. You can mix the Lotus oil with specially made wax or with another oil base in order to create this salve. Lotus Healing Salve promotes calmness and a general feeling of well being.

I can remember a time in my life that I was working for a high volume (and high stress) marketing firm and was seeking out some sort of supplement to take the edge off. I was lucky enough that one of my coworkers was a former direction and herbal therapy expert! She showed me the ropes even before I had ever heard of Herbal Healing Salve. She was the one that introduced me to Lotus as a healing agent and I really think that it quite possibly saved my life! This is the best stress buster in the business! Apply this salve liberally to the arms and chest until you feel better.

Echinacea Salve

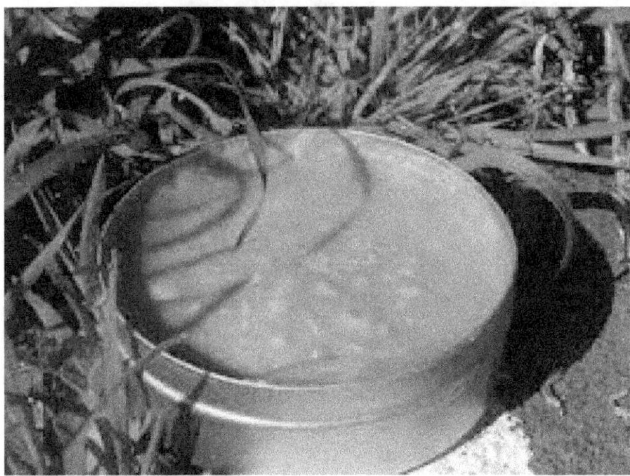

The anti-viral and anti-biotic properties of Echinacea Salve are well known. When this herb is ground into powder you can apply it to your upper body in order to ward off sickness. The aroma of this salve will immediately open your airways benefiting your respiratory system and prolonged use will also begin to greatly enhance your body's immune system as well. This salve is a great boon to your general health, especially in the face of a bad cold or flu episode.

Chamomile Salve

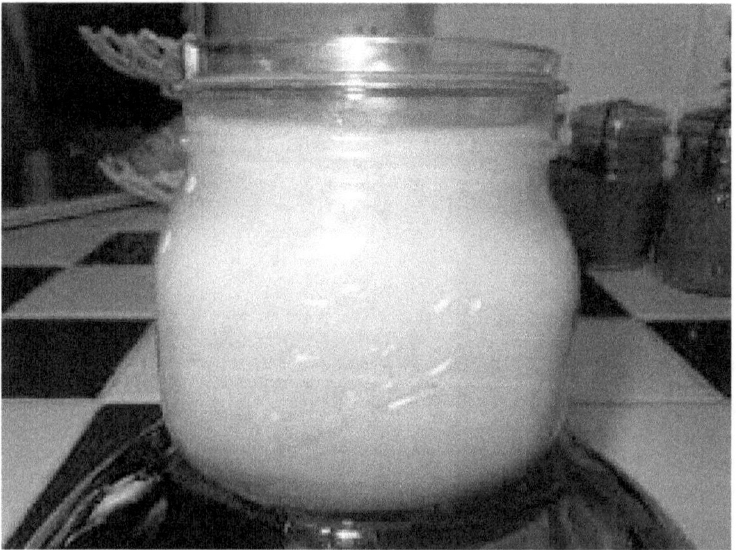

Many people love a good cup of Chamomile tea, well, what about Chamomile Salve? Because the same ingredients that can be found in a cup of Chamomile tea, can be found just as easily in a batch of Chamomile Salve. Take the crushed petals of this flower and blend them together with wax and oil. Store your Chamomile Salve in an airtight plastic container. When this salve is applied to your skin you will immediately start to relax.

And this relaxation is not only skin deep, because what the active ingredients in Chamomile can do is reach down into your very blood vessels, relaxing them and opening them up. Chamomile is a great aid in blood vessel dilation. As a consequence this healing salve is a great aid in controlling blood pressure, doing in many cases what blood pressure pills alone can not. This salve is served well in both powdered form and as oil extract. If you are a already on blood pressure medicine however, you should consult with your doctor first.

Herbal Rose Salve

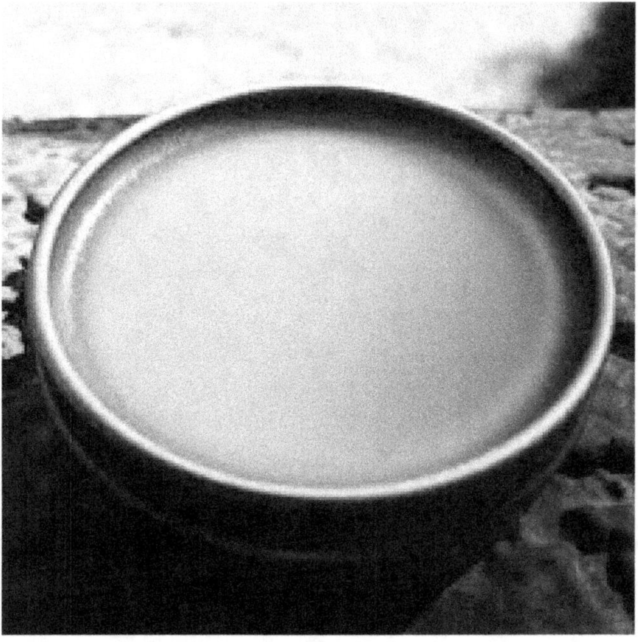

Did you know that Herbal Rose Salve can alleviate stress, depression, and promote sleep for those who experience insomnia? All of these aspects of general wellness and clear states of mind can be facilitated through the special chemicals given off in rose petals.

This is one of the reasons why people feel so good just from smelling the scent of this time honored flower. You ever hear someone say, "It's time to stop and smell the roses?"

Well—given the benefits of this particular healing herb—it certainly couldn't hurt. In order to administer this salve you should mix crushed rose petals with wax and a small base of oil. Store this salve in an airtight container in a cool and dry place. This salve sometimes needs a few days to allow the ingredients to marinate together. So you might want to wait a little bit before application. Once your Herbal Rose Salve is ready to go, use as much as needed.

Rosemary Salve

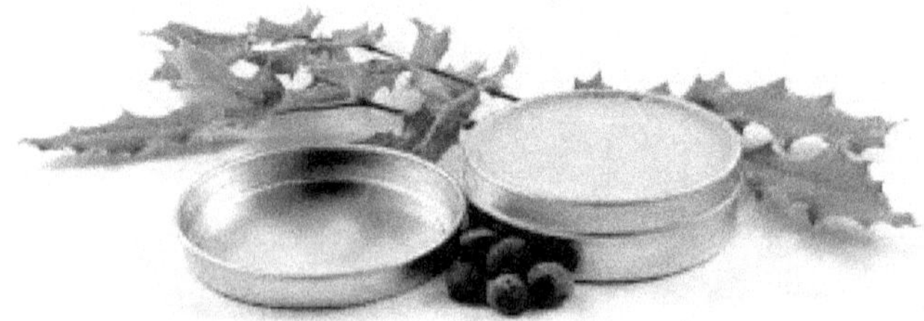

And now that we have covered Herbal Rose Salve, lets take a look at "Rosemary" Salve. Because crushed Rosemary carried in a bit of wax and oil can do wonders for your overall feelings of wellness and health. Rosemary is a detoxing agent and when applied to the body it can work as an exfoliant de-toxing the skin. Rosemary has also been known to raise metabolism and clear up digestive problems.

Once you start a Rosemary regimen you will be amazed at how much more energized you feel. I always keep a tin container of this stuff in a drawer under my desk, and if I ever start feeling a bit sluggish when I'm working I just take a little dab of this stuff and rub it behind my wrists. Within a few minutes I start to feel a healthy rush, and I've got to say, sometimes its even better than coffee!

Chapter 3: Treating Skin Irritation from Cuts, Bites, and Burns

Nothing is worse than a bad sunburn. I used to go to the beach when I was a kid and come back with some of the worst. The same could also be said of waking up with a painful spider bite, rash or cut. In this chapter we set out to show you how the right kind of healing herbal salve can alleviate all of these burdensome issues for you.

Garlic Healing Salve

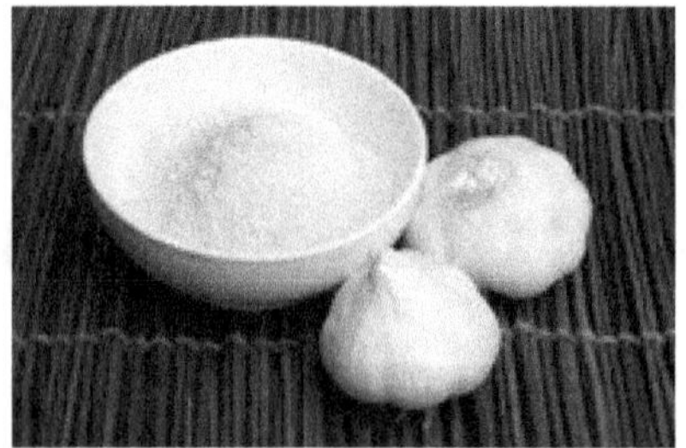

This healing salve works as a significant factor in healing when it comes to cuts and scrapes. Although it is most well known on a piece of Garlic Toast, Garlic Healing Salve can greatly improve the body's own natural healing response. Garlic is an antiseptic and it works as a tool in immunotherapy as well. Garlic can gird the body against colds and flu from just a few ground cloves applied to the skin.

First, grind the Garlic into a fine powder and then add a few drops of regular vegetable oil, thoroughly blending the mixture, this will greatly enhance the potency of the Garlic Healing Salve's effect. If you ever accidentally cut yourself, try to apply this salve immediately. Because it's a salve that can really solve (pun intended) your problems on a major scale.

Aloe Vera Salve

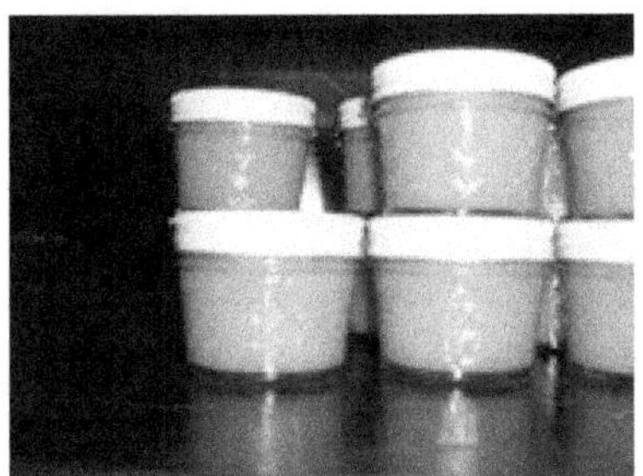

Back when I lived in California I used to swear by this stuff. When Aloe Vera Gel is condensed into a salve it can have tremendous healing potential for the skin. Aloe Vera gel itself can be bought over the counter, then it's just a matter of mixing it with wax and oil. In order to get your own gel however you simply need to cut a leaf off of an Aloe Vera plant, and then take a knife and use it to peel back the surface of the leaf.

It is under here that you will find the deposit of rich gel that every Aloe Vera leaf contains. This can then be mixed with carrier oil. Whenever you get burned just apply your Aloe Vera Salve to where you hurt and you will get relief from your pain. I always keep a jar mason jar of this stuff in my pantry just in case I might need. And I would advise you to do the same. Aloe Vera Salve is a great asset to have no matter what the emergency might be.

Dandelion Herbal Salve

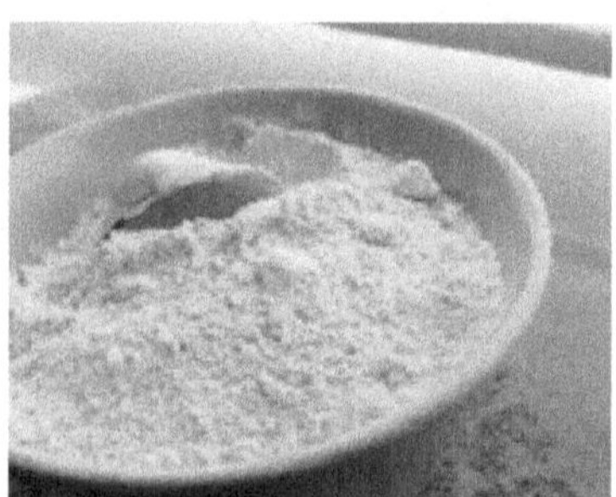

Dandelions are found all over the place—your own yard more than likely has a few—the salve created from this healing herb is spectacular. And besides the healing properties involved, Dandelion roots are known to make for good teas. But to make your dandelion into a suitable salve you should take the whole dandelion and grind it into a fine powder, placing it inside a small airtight container.

This salve can work to alleviate indigestion, and can actually aid insulin function for those who suffer from diabetes. Some diabetics have even managed to go off of their formal treatment and opt for Dandelion treatment instead. This book of course, does not endorse these measures, however and you should always consult your primary physician first. Just thought I would mention that!

In addition to the inroads that Dandelion Herbal Salve has made when it comes to diabetes, Dandelion Herbal Salve also greatly improves the healing of cuts, scrapes and other skin irritation. The active ingredient of this salve has an immediate reaction with the blood platelets that scab over your cuts and sores and promotes a rapid healing. Having this salve around is well worth your effort.

Avocado Bug Bite Salve

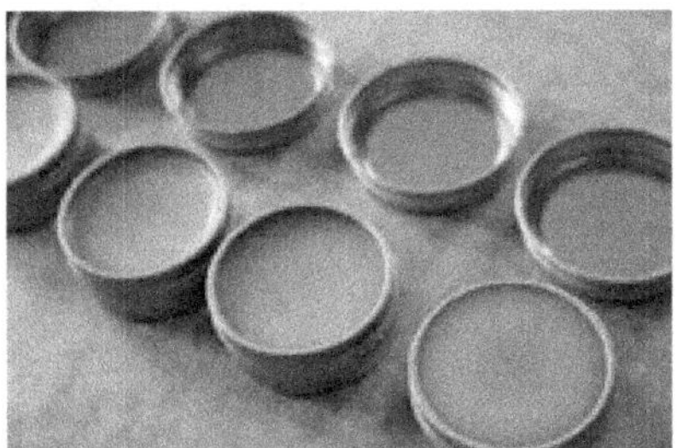

People are amazed when I tell them this, but Avocado works out great for an insect repellant and treatment. It is perhaps better known as an exfoliant for the skin but the active ingredients in Avocado can also take the pain out of a bite or sting. In order to prepare your Avocado Bug Bite Salve, you need to get yourself some beeswax (about half a cup's worth) and mix it with freshly blended Avocado.

After these ingredients are thoroughly blended together place them in a pan and further melt and mold them on medium heat for about 5 minutes as you vigorously stir the contents of the pan. After this dump the contents of the pan into a mason jar, if you have one, and store your Avocado Bug Bite Salve until you really need it. This stuff could last you for years, making it a perfect medical supply to stock up on.

Grapefruit Salve

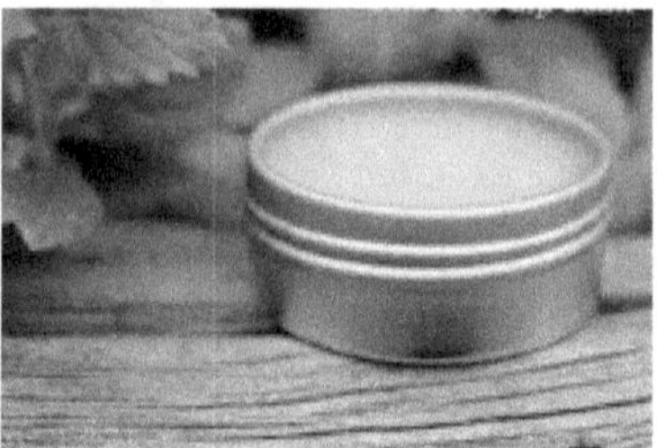

Grapefruit Salve is great for boosting your healing time when it comes to minor cuts and abrasions. It works best as an extracted oil mixed with wax. Put about 20 drops of Grapefruit oil in a pan with some beeswax. Set your burner for medium. Once the contents of your pan have been melted together dump them in a plastic or glass container, seal it, and place in a cool, dry place. This salve works well on most minor cuts and scrapes, just apply it right to the surface of your skin. You should start to feel a slight tingling in your skin. I find that it's best if it is administered at night before you go to sleep, so your cut can heal overnight.

Lemon Healing Salve

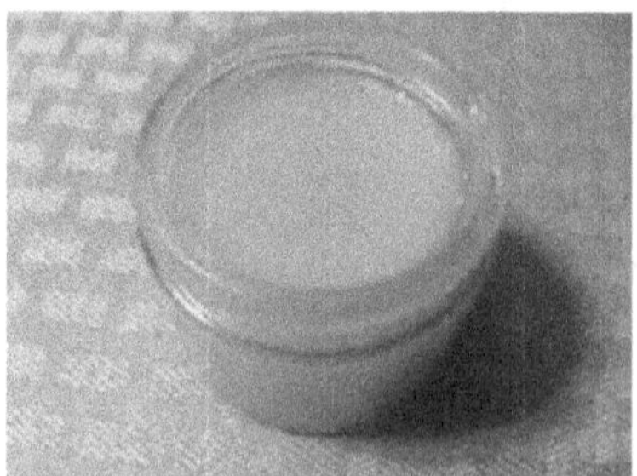

Lemon juice is refreshing in the summertime and so is the salve that can be made from lemon juice. Just take a few drops of this juice and mix it with beeswax. Heat the beeswax up in a pan or in the microwave, melt the ingredients together and then place it in sealable container. This lemon healing salve is a natural antibacterial agent and it works to greatly speed up the entire healing process. Just a small amount of this healing salve applied direct can do you a lot of good.

Lavender Rash Salve

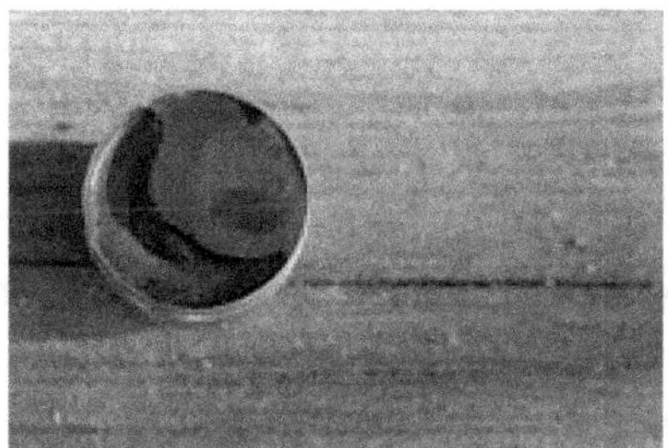

If you have ever suffered from a bad rash after going on a camping trip or just from something you encountered in your own backyard, you know how frustrating such a situation can be. Lavender Rash Salve seeks to solve that. Lavender is best when it is extracted as an essential oil straight from the Lavender plant. Take the oil out mix it with wax and store it in a plastic or glass jar. Apply this Lavender salve directly on your rash so that you can have some relief! Another side benefit of using Lavender as a Salve is that it smells great! Lavender has been used as perfume for many years, and unlike some other Salves that have harsh odors, this one will have you smelling and feeling good!

Ashwagandha Herbal Healing Salve

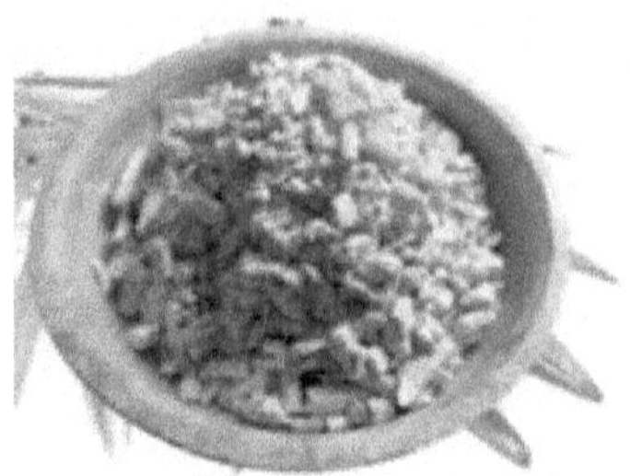

This salve has an amazing ability when it comes to healing flesh wounds. Ashwagandha is a powerful adaptogen that allows you to prep your body for severe physical stress. If you have an open wound on your body you can take this Ashwagandha Herbal Healing Salve and use it to greatly speed up the recovery process. The best way to prepare this salve is to take the herb and grind it into a fine powder. Keep this powder in a safe place and simply rub it on your wound when needed. You should be able to see a marked difference in the healing of your wound in just a few days.

Chapter 4: Some Extra Recipes for the Road!

You never can get enough of a good thing, and when it comes to Healing Herbal Salves this is doubly true. So I thought I would leave you with one more detailed chapter on some of the best salves, with their exact ingredients fully fleshed out.

Soothing Skin Salve

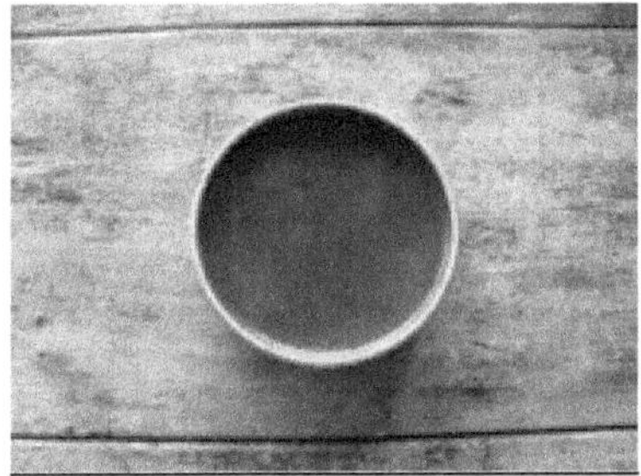

This salve is great for relaxing tight skin around the face and neck. It will also exfoliate and remove any ruptures from present on the surface of the skin.

Here are the exact ingredients:

2 drops of Clove oil

5 drops of Frankincense oil

5 drops of Lavender oil

5 drops of rosemary oil

½ cup of beeswax

Before you get started you will need to get out a good and sturdy double boiler to make it. Place this double boiler in your stove on medium, to medium-high heat. There is no need to bring the contents to a full boil, it just needs to be hot enough for the conents to melt and become well blended together. Once this has been established add the clove oil to the mix. You will notice a pretty heady odor after doing this, if it seems too overpowering just try not to breathe it in directly. After your clove oil begin to deposit the rest of your ingredients as well.

Coconut Smooth Salve

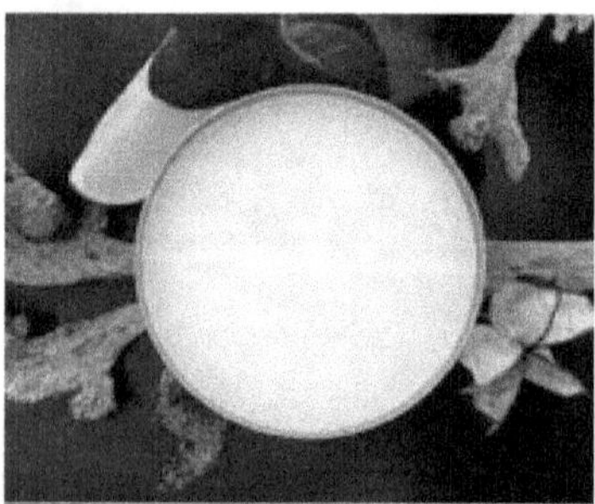

This smooth and refreshing salve will have you feeling good in no time, while smoothing out your skin.

Here are the exact ingredients:

2 drops Coconut oil

½ cup Shea Butter

½ cup Almond oil

Once again, use a double boiler for this recipe, putting it inside the stove at medium-high heat. This time leave it in there just long enough to boil, this typically takes about

4 of 5 minutes. Next, add your drops of Coconut oil. Your coconut oil will be the main base of the salve and will carry the rest of the ingredients. This should then be followed up by adding your half a cup of Shea Butter. Now vigorously stir these contents together. Finally add the half cup of Almond oil and turn off the heat of your stove. Let the whole concoction cool for a bit and then dump it in a glass canning jar.

The Patchouli Happy Hippy Salve

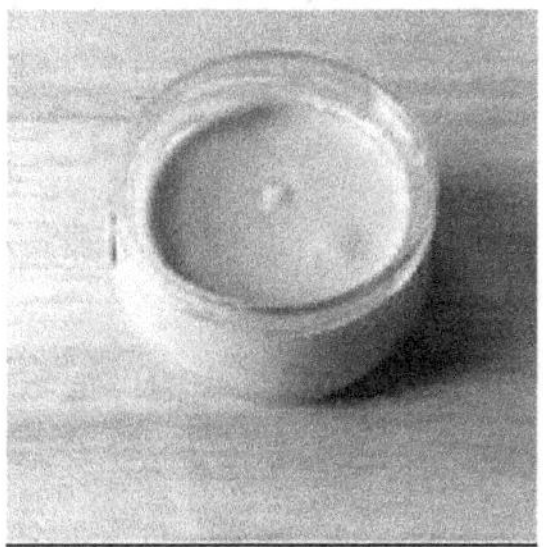

Remember that guy in high school who would come to class absolutely reeking of strong Patchouli? Well now you can smell like him too! All while you help open your airways! I bet you never realized that a bit of Patchouli could be good for your breathing huh? But that is exactly the case! If you suffer from a wide range of breathing problems such as asthma or other issues, The Patchouli Happy Hippy Salve can make you very happy indeed!

Here are the exact ingredients:

7 drops of Chamomile oil

7 drops of Myrrh oil

1 drop of Patchouli oil

3 drops Lavender oil

1/3 cup of Cocoa Butter

¼ cup of water.

Put a regular frying pan on the stove at high heat and add your ¼ cup of water. Now add your 1/3 of a cup of Cocoa Butter to the pan. Next, add your drop of Patchouli oil (Just a drop will do you!). Briefly stir these ingredients together. Now add all of your other ingredients to the mix. Stir them in as well. When you are done add this concoction to a safe canning jar or sealable plastic container.

Geranium Salve

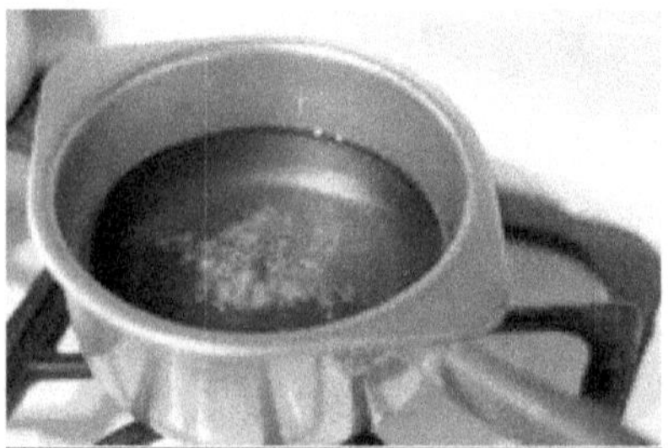

Geranium Salve is great for calming the nerves!

Here are the exact ingredients:

1/3 cup of Beeswax

2 drops of Geranium oil

5 drops of Lavender oil

4 drops of Rosemary oil

Get a hold of that double boiler again, because it's about to go down! On medium heat toss all of your oils into the pan. Stir vigorously. Now add your 1/3 cup of Beeswax and stir it in as well. Allow the mixture to cool and then package it in a jar or plastic container of your choosing. I hope this bonus chapter of extra's has helped key you in to the possibilities!

Conclusion: Getting Back to Nature!

As our society moves further and further away from the basic healing benefits that nature can provide, the kind of life that we can have, begins to deteriorate. This provides us with quite a conundrum since the more a society advances; the healthier it is supposed to be. And yet despite the besting modern medical care, the evidence of this decline is right in front of us in the form of a society that is rapidly becoming obese. An uptake in diabetes and even cancer patients; all indicators that our quality of life is somehow declining, regardless of the medical achievements that have been made over the last 100 years.

For whatever benefits it can give us, the healthcare system is completely mismanaged, the reasons for which can be the basis of an entirely different book, but just in regard to the topic at hand, all you need to know is that the current state of affairs leads to the suffering of our health. In such a conflicted state of affairs, we will find just how much better off we will be if we can just partake of the solutions that nature—quite naturally—provides. I hope that this book has opened your eyes to some of the possibilities out there for us to have a truly healthy and enriching life. Thanks for reading!

FREE Bonus Reminder

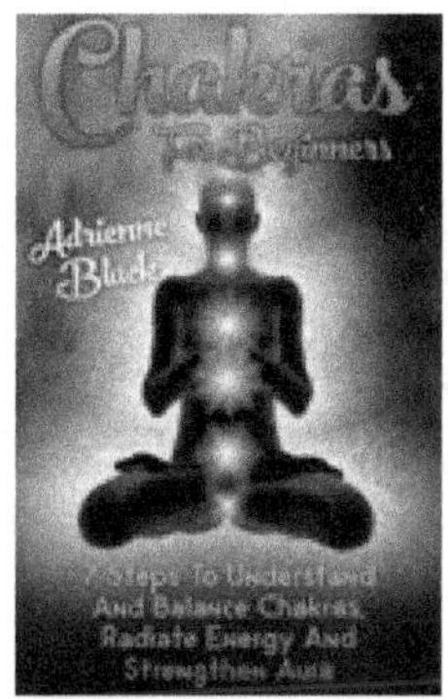

If you have not grabbed it yet, please go ahead and download your special bonus E book *"Chakras for Beginners. 7 Steps To Understand And Balance Chakras, Radiate Energy, And Strengthen Aura"*.

Simply Click the Button Below

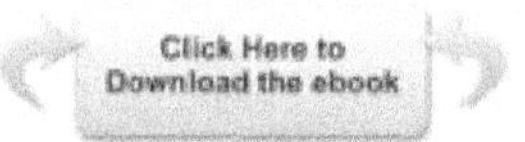

OR Go to This Page

http://lifehacksworld.com/free

BONUS #2: More Free & Discounted Books & Products

Do you want to receive more Free/Discounted Books or Products?

We have a mailing list where we send out our new Books or Products when they go free or with a discount on Amazon. Click on the link below to sign up for Free & Discount Book & Product Promotions.

=> Sign Up for Free & Discount Book & Product Promotions <=

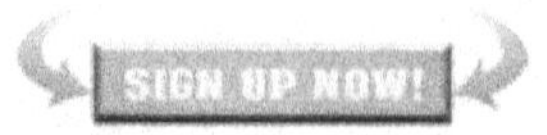

OR Go to this URL

http://zbit.ly/1WBb1Ek

www.ingramcontent.com/pod-product-compliance
Lightning Source LLC
Chambersburg PA
CBHW060823260726
48660CB00003B/1073